My Abbreviated Atlas to Overcoming a Lifetime of Obesity, Shame and Fear

Is This or Was This You?

Table of Contents

Preface

My Abbreviated Atlas to Overcoming a Lifetime of Obesity, Shame and Fear- Is This Or Was This You? was birthed from decades of pain and sadness due to my weight. It wasn't just the "weight" that was my issue. It was how I was treated, which in turn, adversely affected how I viewed myself. Deep down, somehow, I knew I would not only survive, but overcome and demonstrate to others who were at their breaking point of giving up.

I want people to know that giving up should never be an option. We all were born with a purpose inside of us. Some discover "it" early on, some ignore "it," while others, like me, grow and develop into "it" much later. Regarding our mission and life's purpose, There is no deadline. However, once we get there, we just need to focus our energies on the task assigned. I had pondered over sharing my story, and started writing in 2015, two years ago. I had met a really nice, non-judgmental gentleman, who was and is very encouraging of the person I was, as well as the person I was becoming.

I truly hope this book falls into the hands of someone who needs a serious pick-me-up boost to get moving and excited about life. I always say, "It's never too late," but, recently, a few of people near and dear to me have passed away due to weight and health related, possible preventable issues. Maybe my words of hope and honesty can motivate and save just a few. I almost waited until I was stricken with a multitude of illnesses (I was in the early diagnosis phases) before I made a change. Nothing has happened overnight for me to this day, and I am STILL a work in progress! I am not too proud to admit this, and will continue to

grow in grace. Let's grow and shine

together!

Chapter I.

Wow, I am Different!

I can vividly recall as an elementary school

student, dreading physical education, also

known as P.E., or any other outdoor

competitive game or sport, for that matter.

Over 30 plus years ago, there were no

extra-large or fat children in schools--- Well,

maybe myself and one other student out of

the entire grades one through six.

Unsurprisingly, when the bullying began;

this led to shame and embarrassment of my

body very early on in life. No one ever picked me to be on the playground basketball teams, kickball or softball teams, so I made a conscious decision early on that sports just weren't for me. The only outdoor physical activities I enjoyed were jumping double-dutch and bike-riding, which was all fun, but those didn't seem to burn enough calories to propel weight loss. So, guess what happened each year? Yep, you guessed it; I went back to school much bigger after each summer that passed.

Chapter II.

The Shame Must End

Instead of mingling and undressing with the other girls in the general locker room area, I would stand around and wait for a bathroom stall to become available so I could change in private. The other girls didn't seem be bothered by changing around each other, but I saw how small or "normal" they were in size, and wanted to avoid another opportunity to be bullied at all cost. I was even self-conscious about the annual school scoliosis screening, and had my Mother write a note to the teacher that I preferred to have my test alone and

not in the main room with the other girls.
Of course a young girl's brain space wasn't
supposed to be saturated and consumed by
such trepidation, but, sadly, mine was. Fast
forward 30 years, and I'm still plagued with
obesity. This became the new term (and I
was a Spelling Bee winner who'd never
seen this word back then) for being **REALLY**
fat, but was unheard of decades ago. The
physical and emotional woes that came
with being super-sized had become a
barrier between me and my experiencing
the great things life had to offer. At age 35, I
was working in healthcare, and with
thorough research, I made a life-changing

decision to have weight loss surgery. At that point, I had eaten, cried and stressed myself up to nearly 400 pounds. Many popular diet programs, pills and fads were attempted, but none of them ever yielded the results to keep me motivated. I can even recall sharing an office with two other ladies (both who are very nice and are still my friends to this very day), praying each day that my office chair wouldn't break. To live in such paranoia is by no means living. I sit here in my little office today, humbled and overwhelmed with gratitude and excitement, as it always seemed to be the "small *normal* things" that I could not relate to for the majority of my life. Today, I have no excuses for not reaching, stretching, striving and telling my story. I hope to save someone- at least one person, letting them see that they're not alone. I can no longer be silenced by pain, fear and regret.

I'M READY TO COME OUT! I AM READY TO FINALLY FREE MYSELF!!!

Chapter III.

The Start of Something New

On the morning of my weight loss surgery, I had God and my sister with me- that was it.

There was no more fear or pain that could have outweighed the suffering and torment I had already been afflicted with.

I was ready and willing to see what the light would reveal at the end of the tunnel. My mind and spirit were at peace, and it was only up, up, up, from here, I felt.

Trust me; I had even shocked myself, as my history had shown that I could not succeed at weight loss or much else in my life. Each day thereafter came with a new discovery, a new milestone, which gave me continued hope. Learning to have faith in God, believing in myself, and knowing I could help someone prevented me from throwing in the towel many a day. Of course it also helped that I was completely horrified of what people would say about my dead, obese corpse. I know, what kind of weird thinker was I?

I discovered that quitting in the middle of the "game of life" was not an option. Though I had pondered and conjured up ways to end my life, they had all failed. After all, they had to, so I could live to fulfill my passion, attributed to my life of pain. My assignment on planet Earth hadn't even begun. I woke up each day, knowing that I had done myself and others a *major solid* by choosing to live and not give in.

After the first few months of my new body change, I decided it was time to join a gym to propel my weight loss and increase my functionality. I found a facility that, not only had the set-up of what I needed, but one that was size-friendly and non-intimidating. Yes, it matters what the atmosphere is when it comes to feeling comfortable working out. Being a former choir singer, let's just say, I had found me a choir that would let me sing in it—MAJOR SCORE!!! My gym was a hospital managed facility, and I joined after the initial tour! I was in—

hook, line, and sinker! Of course, I thought at times I was the biggest, fattest, most ginormous monstrosity of a human, but that didn't stop me. I was in autopilot mode. There were days that I physically and mentally ached to no end. Hey, no pain, no gain, right? Well, in my case, no loss of lbs... I didn't want to revert to my years of painkiller popping. I would take anywhere from six to ten pain pills just to get through my routine activities of daily living. I guess I was an addict in more ways than one. Luckily and thankfully, my gym had a heated therapy pool and hot tub that made all my workouts have a happy ending. I literally felt like a baby learning to walk for the very first time. I increased my time and intensity in very small increments. The days I couldn't make it to gym, I worked out at home doing free weights, therapy bands, stretching in bed or my exercise bike when I could. I was determined to win at this! I didn't always live by this mantra, but it's undoubtedly a good one to follow:

You are entitled to take up whatever amount of space necessary for you to function and thrive in this world.

I wish I could yell this on a bullhorn on every mountaintop and in every valley. No matter your size, sickness, disability or difference in appearance compared to others, this basic principle *must* reside within your brain and spirit.

Also, **"You are not the key focal point of everyone around you, believe it or not."** Remember, people may stare for a moment, but don't let stares and whispers deter your mission.

Chapter IV.

Maintaining Confidence Along the Way

Once you begin to see the results, though big or small, give yourself credit and hold on to your happy. Don't ever let it slip from you. You will need each ounce to propel you to the next level coming.

There's always a surprise around the corner. Trying on clothes in smaller sizes, buying belts for the first time, watching the notches move further down, getting in/out of your vehicle with ease, buckling your seat belt, flying on a plane for the first time, flying with no seatbelt extender, etc. are all reasons to celebrate those small successes or non-scale victories. I can't list them all here, but you get the idea.

Find something about yourself that you like.

I know this is not an easy request. You may not be in love with your body, but there has to be something, some part of you that you are at least somewhat fond of—Whether it's your beautiful hands, legs, toes, smile, eyes, just something. Look long and hard in the mirror and begin to respect and love on yourself. Do this exercise daily, because you're worth it. Appreciate the life you've been given, and the opportunity to become better. As with anything, this will take time, practice and patience, but is indeed possible. I can still hear my Mother telling me, "Pam, stop slouching, shoulders back, chin-up!" My Mother swore that by having good posture, you've automatically slimmed yourself down by 10-15 pounds.

What can I do now that I wasn't able to do in the past? What can I look forward to?

These two questions are relevant to attaining the confidence needed to get from where you are to your destiny. If there are things that I desire to aspire and achieve, I immediately make an effort to go into "grateful mode." Being grateful for the positive changes allow me to have a glimmer, or ray of hope for this awesome life I've been given.

Chapter V.

Healthy is not a Size

Is being healthy necessarily a dress or pant size? Healthy can be measured by how you feel when you complete daily tasks, chores and challenges, in addition to having a good medical checkup. Do you become winded after getting out of your car to pump gas? Are you able to walk around the stores and shop without leg or knee pain? Does housecleaning put you in asthmatic attack mode? Shoot, how about when you simply drop something on the floor, and have to pick it up? I spent decades thinking I was the only one with these issues. Surely no one had it as bad as me, right? Well, today I know better for sure.

Chapter VI.

I Am not a Garbage Disposal

The purpose of a garbage disposal is to dispose of waste, be it leftovers, scraps, etc., that is no longer wanted or desired. I remember the years I had no concept or concern of the quantity and quality of food I was consuming. There were late night runs to the local convenience stores (which were not so convenient in calories and pounds, but I was delusional) for ice cream sundaes with extra fudge, and birthday cake when it was no one's birthday that I knew of. Shoot, I would even have the cake labeled to read, "Happy Birthday" or "Congratulations" just to make it look good to the cashier at the check-out. Of course I could go on with the tales of poisoning and intoxicating my body, but, again, I know I wasn't the only one.

Knowing and finally discovering the benefits of eating healthier is a feeling like no other. From the glow of my skin, to the ease of my output (TMI I know), I can say that every new positive change I've made has been

more than worth it!

It's great when others notice the

physical changes in you, but feeling them

from the inside out is

 PRICELESS!

Chapter VII.

Don't Be Afraid to try New Things

Fear can tend to get the best of us

when all we know is things being done

one particular way. Being resistant to

the thought of experimenting with

activities, or even trying new foods

can be intimidating or horrifying in

some instances. I think back to the

times when I was petrified to be seen

in a bathing suit. Then I (once again)

would quickly remind myself that

everyone is here for the same reason

and purpose, which is for health,

wellness, edification or recreation.

Why should I continue missing out on

swimming when I love the water, too?

When trying to find things that may fit

you when you're just getting started,

look online, or don't be afraid to ask

others of similar body size/type where

they shop. People generally don't

mind sharing helpful information, and

may even be flattered that you'd ask

them. Once you find something to

wear that makes you somewhat

comfortable in- don't stop there!

Get started and **DON'T LOOK BACK** at those days of sedentary inactivity! Moving your body is not an option. A body in motion will almost always want be in motion. This is so cliché, but you will crave and reap the endless benefits of physical activity in no time! In this journey of health and wellness, we don't always know what we need; but, with each positive choice, we gain more knowledge, strength and power!

Chapter VIII.

Hacks to Utilize in the Weight Loss Journey

Now, I would be remiss if I didn't dedicate a section of this self-help roadmap to weight loss hacks that got/are still getting me through this life journey. These are not listed in any specific order, please note:

- Believe in yourself. No one will think highly of you without you first doing so.

- Surround yourself with positive people. This can be online support, friends, family, mates, etc.

- Surround yourself with people who will keep and hold you accountable by being honest with you when you don't want to hear it.

- Never forget how far you've come. Always keep a bitter herb for reflection- Old pictures, journals, notes to yourself, etc.

- Seek the advice and mentorship of someone you trust (personally or professionally).

- Accept a compliment and don't challenge or reject it.

- Engage in social activities, groups, projects, etc.

- Be an example, a good friend and offer kind words, support and motivation to others in need.

- Hone in on something you like about yourself and seek out ways to accentuate and showcase your attributes appropriately.

- **BE GRATEFUL**. Remember, there are no carbon copies of you. Not one!+! No one was ever meant to be you, and you were never meant to be anyone but you. After all, takes all kind to make the world 'go round.'

- Don't look down, demean or frown upon someone who may not be where you are in their journey. Keep in mind; you weren't always the person you are today!

This may sound cliché, but,
IF I CAN FIND HOPE, SO CAN YOU!
You are worth the sacrifice and self-investment of health! You have what it takes to be great!
I'M ROOTING FOR YOU ALL THE WAY!!!!!!
-Pam ☺